It's Not Just Menopause; It's Your Thyroid!

25 Thyroid and Hashimoto's Truths That Explain Why You Feel So Lousy, Drowsy, Exhausted, and Lost!

By Dr. Joni Labbe, DC, CCN, DCCN

Disclaimer

This book represents the sole opinions of the author, and is not intended to be a substitute for working with a medical or healthcare professional. It is not intended to treat or diagnose. The self-help aspects of this book do not replace professional treatment and should not be considered as diagnosis or treatment of any kind.

The names and all identifying information of the women who generously contributed to this book have been changed in order to respect their privacy.

Table of Contents

Introduction – Who Says the Second Half of Your Life Can't be the Best Half?

If you are reading this book it is almost certainly because you feel like you just aren't YOU anymore. Somehow over the last few years your body has gone from being your best friend to being a prison…a run-down, barely functioning prison at that!

Many of the women who have walked into my health clinic over the past decade list off a whole reel of symptoms. They tell me that they feel like some invisible force has vacuumed up all of their energy, yet they still toss and turn at night. They wonder why all the hair on their head is migrating to their chin, why their skin is so dry and flakey, and why even the strictest diet isn't budging those ten extra pounds. My clients also lean in and confidentially admit that they are as dry as the Mojave Desert "down there" and never feel "in the mood" with their spouses anymore.

Every one of these women have been to the doctor. In fact, many of my clients run out of fingers and start using toes when they tick off all the doctors and professionals they've seen. They've been told that their blood tests are normal and that their symptoms are simply the result of aging. Some were handed synthetic thyroid hormones that work for a while before the symptoms return. Others receive prescriptions for anxiety medication. Friends and family members subtly (and sometimes not so subtly) suggest that it's all in the woman's head; that she is overreacting and just needs to get used to it.

Does this experience sound familiar? If it does, then you're reading the right book.

The truth is that women don't wilt like flowers after menopause. If you don't feel like yourself, then something truly is wrong inside your body, and it needs to be addressed. I wrote this book for all the women who come to my clinic as a last, desperate attempt to feel better.

Currently, traditional medicine is very good at addressing acute injuries and illnesses, but it is not structured to identify and manage imbalances within the body that lead to a cascade of mysterious symptoms. Traditional medicine focuses on sewing up gashes and handing out medication to dampen symptoms.

I practice a different sort of healing, known as functional medicine. Functional medicine looks at the whole person – the story that their symptoms are telling – and attempts to treat the cause of the symptoms, rather than just mute the symptoms themselves. In most cases, the culprit is not a single thing, but rather a host of imbalances that each affects the others. We must carefully shift the body back into balance using a variety of methods, including diet, supplementation, exercise, and more.

This is exactly what I've helped hundreds of women do for over twenty years at my health clinic down in San Diego. I am a board certified clinical nutritionist and chiropractor, and I am also a follower of my own protocol. In 2007 I discovered that I had Hashimoto's disease, (more on this a little later), after doing the same testing on myself that I suggest for all my clients. This realization was a huge wakeup call for me. It set me on the path of discovering how to help women like myself who felt like they were falling apart and weren't getting the answers that they were looking for from their doctors.

This book, *It's Not Just Menopause,* is an opening salvo to help women understand where their symptoms are coming from. Knowledge is power. In this book, I set out to tell you the 25 most important truths that you need to know about autoimmune conditions – things you will almost never hear at your doctor's office. Remember, most doctors want to move patients in and out of their exam rooms as fast as possible. They may do blood tests, but if they don't see any red flags, they'll send you out the door with a wave and possibly a prescription for Prozac. You need answers, and you can start getting them here!

This short book is not meant to be a comprehensive guide to autoimmune disease, hypothyroidism, or functional medicine protocols. This is simply a start, a first look inside your body. If the content in this book really speaks to you, I strongly suggest becoming a member of the Mojo Girlfriend's community I created at **www.MojoGirlfriends.com** and picking up a copy of my book, *Why Is Mid-Life Mooching Your Mojo?* In this book, I go into much more detail about autoimmunity and how to manage conditions like Hashimoto's, hypothyroidism, and other autoimmune disorders.

For now, my beautiful new friend, know that you are not Lazy, Crazy, or Finished! Arm yourself with knowledge and with truth.

Enjoy!

Joni Labbe, DC, CCN, DCCN

Thyroid Truth #1: Normal Lab Tests Don't Mean That Your Thyroid is Normal

Susan has always prided herself on her focus and energy. It's how she became a VP of her company and raised three kids along the way. The problem is that this powerful, driven, and balanced lady hasn't felt like any of those things over the last month. In fact, she's been a total wreck – unable to sleep at night and exhausted and groggy in the morning. Sometimes she zones out at meetings or feels her heart start racing for no reason as she drives to work. The hair in the drain and extra pounds on the scale aren't doing a thing for her self-esteem.

What the heck is happening? Is this what aging is supposed to feel like, or is something wrong?

Susan finally takes off work and visits her doctor's office. After describing her symptoms, Susan's doctor suggests a blood test to measure her thyroid. The doctor explains that the thyroid is a butterfly-shaped gland that sits at the front of the neck and releases thyroid hormones. These hormones play a big role in regulating the body's metabolism. If the thyroid isn't releasing enough hormones, or the proper balance of hormone, that could explain Susan's exhaustion, brain fog, and other symptoms.

The day after Susan's blood test, the doctor calls to tell Susan that the test came back, and her thyroid is 4.5, on the high side of normal. Susan is relieved to know that her thyroid isn't malfunctioning but also flummoxed. If her thyroid isn't out of whack, what is causing her symptoms? Will she ever get better, or is this her new reality?

Unfortunately, Susan's story is all too common. I have met so many women who go to their doctors only to be assured that their blood tests are normal, when in fact "normal" doesn't actually mean "normal" at all!

The current medical standards that define normal thyroid function are incredibly broad. If a client's level of Thyroid Stimulating Hormone (TSH) is between 0.35 to 5.0, the test will be considered normal.

In fact, the optimal level of TSH is 1.8 to 3.0. This is the range at which a person will feel healthy, energetic, and focused. You may be "functional" with a TSH below 1.8, the same way you can be "functional" by eating just 1,200 calories a day, but you will not be optimal.

When we look at health, we need to go beyond diagnosing severe illness and focus on supporting true health. Susan may not be in a wheelchair or completely immobilized, but she is certainly not well. Her TSH indicates that her thyroid is not creating enough thyroid hormone, which means she is suffering from hypothyroidism.

If Susan just accepts her doctor's diagnosis, she may never realize where her symptoms are coming from until her thyroid continues to deteriorate to the point where she becomes sick enough that her blood tests will raise red flags. We don't want to wait until Susan gets to that point!

"Functional" is not good enough for me, and don't let it be good enough for you. Even if your doctor has told you that your blood tests are normal, now you know better.

Thyroid Truth #2: Your Hypothyroidism Might be Caused by Hashimoto's

On most occasions your immune system is your friend. In fact, your immune system really deserves to be among your best friends. When a virus invades your body, your white blood cells rush to the scene to defeat the enemy and defend your lovely self.

However, in certain situations, your immune system can get tricked or accidentally mistake something good for something bad. In fact, this is exactly what happens in the case of Hashimoto's thyroiditis. Never heard of it? You aren't alone.

I bet you have heard of hypothyroidism. This is a condition where the thyroid produces low amounts of thyroid stimulating hormone (TSH). Since the TSH helps regulate the body's metabolism, a lack of TSH is like adding water to your car's tank instead of gasoline. Those who suffer from hypothyroidism often feel exhausted, gain weight, experience brain fog, and basically feel lousy most of the time, like Susan.

If you have hypothyroidism or know someone who does, it's likely that the cause of your condition is Hashimoto's disease. In fact, Hashimoto's is the number one cause of low thyroid or hypothyroidism in the United States. Though it can affect men and women of all ages, it is found most prominently in post-menopausal women.

What is Hashimoto's, and why does it lead to hypothyroidism?

Hashimoto's occurs when your immune system mistakes TSH for an intruder. For example, let's say that your immune system is a huge Boston Red Sox fan, which means, of course, that it hates the New York Yankees with a vengeance. New York Yankees fans tend to wear navy blue baseball caps, so your immune system decides to attack anyone wearing a navy blue ball cap. Here comes your thyroid, minding its own business, proudly wearing a navy blue San Diego Padres cap. Your immune system can't tell the difference between the Yankees hat and the Padres hat. All it sees is a navy blue cap, which means – ATTACK!

When someone has Hashimoto's disease, their immune system often attacks the thyroid, which results in lower functioning, less thyroid hormone, and all the lousy symptoms that make you feel like you're falling apart.

When you have Hashimoto's, you don't have just a "thyroid" problem, you have an "autoimmune" problem! This is an important distinction, because the thyroid hormones that doctors commonly prescribe to hypothyroid patients do nothing to manage their Hashimoto's. All they do is mask the symptoms by providing your body with synthetic thyroid. If you have a leak in your gas tank, adding more gas will help your car keep running, but it won't fix the leak!

Unfortunately, many doctors don't even test for Hashimoto's disease! They see a high TSH level on your blood test (which tells them that your thyroid isn't functioning well) and prescribe synthetic hormone to help address your symptoms. That's not good enough! When you have an immune system problem, the solution is to heal your immune system, not just load your body up with synthetic hormone. As you'll learn as you read further, I believe it's time to stop just putting more gas in the car and start looking at ways to fix the leak.

Thyroid Truth #3: Your Doctor Probably Isn't Running the Right Blood Tests on You

Hashimoto's disease is a nasty little trickster dupes your immune system into attacking your thyroid, which, over time, results in hypothyroidism. As we just learned, Hashimoto's is the leading cause of hypothyroidism in the United States and is particularly common among post-menopausal women.

You'd think that when you walk into your doctor's office and explain that you've been feeling exhausted, anxious, and forgetful for no reason, your doctor would immediately run a battery of blood tests to look for Hashimoto's.

In most cases, you'd be wrong! Many doctors will only run a test that looks at the level of TSH in your blood. This number will tell your doctor whether your thyroid is working within normal ranges (which you now know itself is a misnomer) but NOT whether or not you have Hashimoto's.

Okay, so you're thinking, *Why in the heck doesn't my doctor look for Hashimoto's? Is it impossible to find or something?*

Doctors usually don't look for Hashimoto's, because they typically respond the same way whether you have Hashimoto's or not. They see low thyroid functioning and prescribe synthetic thyroid to treat the problem. In some cases, your symptoms may go away for a time, but there's a big problem with this protocol…It doesn't actually solve the problem!

Like I mentioned in the last section, if your gas tank is leaking, the solution isn't to simply add more gas to the tank, it's to fix the leak. In order to fix the leak, you have to know that the leak actually exists.

Hashimoto's is not impossible to find. In fact, your doctor just needs to run a blood test that looks for special antibodies called TPO and TGB antibodies. If these guys show up on your test results, then you have an autoimmune thyroid, otherwise known as – Hashimoto's disease.

Once you've identified the cause of your hypothyroid symptoms, you can start to figure out ways to calm your immune system down so it doesn't keep throwing punches at your thyroid. We will look at some of these solutions later in the book. First though, I'll answer the question – How can I tell if I have an autoimmune condition?

Thyroid Truth #4: Three Ways to Tell if Your Immune System is Attacking Your Body

If you have Hashimoto's, your immune system has mistaken your thyroid for an intruder and is attacking your poor little gland. This is why you feel exhausted all the time, like a car with water in the gasoline tank. Your thyroid just can't give you all the thyroid hormones that you need to keep your metabolism revved up.

How do you know if you have Hashimoto's disease and that your thyroid isn't just out of whack on its own? The easiest way to know is to have your blood tested for TPO and TGB antibodies. When these guys show up on your blood panel, it means your immune system is in full attack mode.

Even before you come in for blood tests, there are common symptoms that can indicate an autoimmune thyroid. Here are three surefire clues that your immune system is beating up on your thyroid:

Clue One: You Already Have An Autoimmune Disorder

Do you suffer from psoriasis, rheumatoid arthritis, ulcerative colitis, Sjogren's syndrome, scleroderma, or lupus? If so, then your immune system is already attacking your body. Once you have one autoimmune disorder, you are at a much higher risk of getting another. (When it rains, it pours!)

Clue Two: Your Symptoms Wax and Wane

When you suffer from a regular illness, like a cold, your symptoms grow worse for a few days and then slowly get better until you kick the cold for good. An autoimmune disease doesn't work that way. Your immune system responds again and again when it senses intruders, which results in symptoms that come and go. If you've gotten used to having "good days" and "bad days," you may have an autoimmune disorder.

Clue Three: You Take Lots Of Supplements

I can't tell you how many new clients bring in bags filled with their supplements to my office. Autoimmune diseases usually cause a multitude of symptoms that may not seem interconnected. For instance, you may combat your weariness with green tea, take glucosamine to help with stiff joints, St. John's Wort to help relieve your anxiety, and ginko biloba to clear your brain fog.

It's easy to see each symptom as its own unique problem with its own solution, but in reality, they might all stem from the same root – an autoimmune disease.

If any of these three clues is familiar to you, as in, "That's totally me!" then I strongly recommend getting your blood for TPO and TGB antibodies. You don't actually have to go to your doctor to have these blood tests done. You can visit a private lab if you are willing to pay for the blood test out of pocket. Since, as you now know many doctors treat an autoimmune condition like Hashimoto's by just managing the symptoms (not the cause), you may be more comfortable working with a private thyroid specialists. I often refer my clients to private labs near them. When the results of the blood tests arrive, we review the results together in person if they are local or over the phone if they live out of state.

If you suspect that you have an autoimmune condition, I bet one of your top questions is, *Why me?* Next we look at some of the most common causes of autoimmune disorders.

Thyroid Truth #5: Your Autoimmune Disease is Caused by Genetics and the Environment

When a woman comes into my office complaining of a truckload of symptoms – from exhaustion to thinning hair, dry skin, low libido, and weight gain – I always suggest a blood panel. More often than not, the blood panel reveals an autoimmune disease, usually Hashimoto's.

When I give the client the results of the test, her question is almost always the same. "How did I get an autoimmune disease?"

The answer is that autoimmune diseases are caused by a combination of genetics and environmental triggers. Think of it as a light switch inside your DNA that can remain off or be flipped on.

Genetics

The light switch is the genetic component. If your grandmother or mother had an autoimmune condition, such as psoriasis, rheumatoid arthritis, lupus, etc…, then you have a higher-than-average risk of also developing an autoimmune disorder. In other words, you have an autoimmune light switch in your DNA, which environmental factors can flip on.

Environmental Factors

Our environment is filled with chemicals that affect the way the body works and how certain parts of our DNA expresses itself. The buildup of harmful chemicals in our body can flip disease switches in the DNA, causing all sorts of trouble, including autoimmune disorders. What are some of the environmental factors that might flip on your autoimmune light switch? Here are just four:

Cigarettes: Over 519 chemicals reside inside a single cigarette. When you smoke, you invite these chemicals directly into your body through your lungs. These chemicals can wreak havoc on your body and trigger your autoimmune disease.

BPA: You've probably heard about bisphenol A, or BPA in the news over the last few years. It's gotten a pretty bad rep, and with good reason. This chemical, found in many plastics, is extremely bad for your thyroid health. Luckily, the word is getting out about BPA, and many responsible manufacturers are eliminating it from their products.

Rocket fuel: Yes, you read that correctly, I wrote rocket fuel! You may ask, "How can there possibly be rocket fuel inside of me? It's not like I drink the stuff for breakfast." Some surprising studies have shown that 30 to 40 percent of women in America have trace amounts of rocket fuel in their body. Rocket fuel can leech into groundwater and stay there for a very long time.

Iodine: Forget everything you've heard about how iodine strengthens the thyroid. In fact, the opposite is true. Iodine is one of the BIGGEST triggers for

Hashimoto's disease. If you even suspect that you might have an autoimmune disorder, you need to break up with your iodine supplements permanently!

Let's take a closer look at exactly why iodine is so bad for your thyroid in the next section.

Thyroid Truth #6: Iodine is Not Your Thyroid's Friend!

Let's say that you walk into a health food store and tell the manager, "I have a thyroid condition. What can I do to help my thyroid?" The manager will probably cheerfully hand you a bottle of iodine supplements. The manager means well, she really does, but iodine is about the worst thing she could have put into your hands.

Despite popular belief, taking iodine can actually make your thyroid condition worse.

It's easy to understand why the confusion occurs. Iodine is vital to thyroid function. It is a major stimulator for an enzyme called TPO which plays a role in the production of thyroid stimulating hormone. If you suffer from hypothyroidism, then your thyroid isn't producing enough thyroid hormone. In this situation, it seems to make sense to take iodine. You need thyroid stimulating hormone and that's what iodine helps your body produce.

Unfortunately, this logic doesn't factor in autoimmune conditions, like Hashimoto's disease. When you have Hashimoto's, your immune system mistakes thyroid hormone for an intruder and attacks the thyroid. The more thyroid hormone in your body, the more the immune system attacks.

My good friend, Dr. Datis Kharrazian, author of *Why Do I Still Have My Thyroid Symptoms?* compares taking iodine supplements to throwing gasoline onto a fire. Your immune system will go haywire as the iodine stimulates your thyroid to produce more hormones. Some people who take iodine supplements show symptoms of an overactive thyroid, while others show elevated levels of TPO antibodies on their blood panel, (which means that the immune system is attacking the thyroid), even though they experience no symptoms.

If you even suspect that you might have an autoimmune thyroid condition, then stop taking iodine immediately and avoid foods that are heavy in iodine, like seaweed, yogurt, milk, and eggs. Also, look on the back of the bottle of your multivitamin. If you see iodine in the list, then it's time to take a new multivitamin.

The manager at the health food store means well, but she probably doesn't have a medical background. Now that you know the truth about iodine, let's look at another big no, no – Tyrosine.

Thyroid Truth #7: Tyrosine Doesn't Help Your Thyroid Either!

Remember that helpful manager at the health food store who is ready to load your basket up with iodine supplements to help your thyroid? Now that you know that iodine is one of the worst things you can put into your body if you have an autoimmune thyroid disorder, you can politely decline the iodine supplements. So, what is the next supplement the manager might suggest?

My bet is on tyrosine. Just like iodine, tyrosine plays an integral role in thyroid hormone production, and just like iodine, it is not something you want to take if you have a low performing thyroid.

Tyrosine may actually suppress thyroid activity. In fact, you won't find a single study that shows that tyrosine can increase the production of thyroid hormone.

What happens instead is that tyrosine will increase adrenal hormones, like epinephrine and norepinephrine, which create a jittery feeling. You may experience a strange, floaty kind of high. While this might sound intriguing, what's actually happening is that the tyrosine is over-stimulating the adrenals glands and causing a stress response. This isn't good for your thyroid or your health!

The moral of this story is that the manager or clerk at

your local health food store is probably not the best resource for your supplementation recommendations. Instead, you really need to be have a blood panel performed so that a thyroid specialist can review the results and determine what is actually happening in your body. Once you and your practitioner understand what is going on, you can begin to address the problem with real solutions and then test again to see if they are working.

Thyroid Truth #8: Your Low Thyroid Could Actually be Anemia

We know that Hashimoto's disease is the number on cause of hypothyroidism in the United States. However, that doesn't mean it's the only cause of hypothyroidism. The thyroid can be affected by a number of different things, including other hormones.

When a client comes to me with symptoms of hypothyroidism, and their blood tests don't show the usual antibodies that suggest an autoimmune condition, the next most likely suspect is anemia.

Anemia means that you either have a low number of red blood cells or that your red blood cells don't contain enough hemoglobin, an iron-rich protein that helps blood cells carry oxygen throughout the body.

Oxygen is life. It fuels your muscles, brain, and organs. When you are low on red blood cells or hemoglobin, your body isn't getting enough oxygen. Think about how tired you'd feel if you could only fill your lungs up halfway with each breath. That's what's happening to your muscles and brain when you have anemia. As a result, you'll often feel weak, cold, shaky, and mentally dull. Do these symptoms sound familiar? These are many of the same symptoms of hypothyroidism!

The common "cure" for anemia is iron supplementation, but that isn't always the right solution. Some forms of anemia don't respond to iron supplements, and they can actually make the condition worse by breaking down red blood cells. Too much iron in the body can be toxic (even worse than mercury or other heavy metals).

When I encounter a client who does not have an autoimmune condition, I immediately test for anemia, blood sugar, gut/liver function, and fatty acid metabolism. Usually the culprit is in one of these categories.

If you worry that you have anemia, or if you already know you have the condition and haven't been responding to iron supplements, it's time to get a blood panel and try a different solution.

Thyroid Truth #9: Prolactin May be Causing Your Low Thyroid

Now we know that hypothyroidism isn't always caused by an autoimmune condition, like Hashimoto's disease. There are other reasons why your thyroid might be clocking out early every day and leaving you with less thyroid than you need to feel good. One reason is too little prolactin.

Think of your body as a sensitive ecosystem balanced by optimal levels of hormones, chemicals, proteins, and even bacteria. As long as everything stays in balance, you feel energetic, clear-headed, and ready to take on the world. But if one piece of the equation falls out of whack, the entire ecosystem can suffer.

Prolactin, made by the pituitary gland, is one of the many hormones swimming around inside your body. It is especially active during pregnancy, where it helps women make breast milk for their future bundle of joy.

Hormones interact with each other. Too much or too little of one can dampen or increase another. Progesterone and dopamine balance prolactin. When someone suffers from a dopamine or progesterone deficiency, this basically leaves the door open for progesterone to go hog wild inside your body. As a result, the higher levels of prolactin will put stress on the pituitary gland.

What does this have to do with thyroid function? Well, the pituitary gland is usually a great multitasker. It doesn't just create prolactin, it also produces thyroid stimulating hormone (TSH), which as its name implies, tells the thyroid to make thyroid hormone. Think of TSH as the "giddy-up" for the thyroid to produce the thyroid hormone your body needs to stay metabolically balanced.

When the pituitary gland has its metaphorical hands full making excess prolactin, it can't make as much TSH, which means less giddy-up for your thyroid and less thyroid hormone in your body.

When you feel weak and sluggish, can't lose weight, experience thinning hair, and notice any of the many other symptoms of a low thyroid, it's time to come in for testing. Just testing for low thyroid isn't enough. You and your thyroid specialist need to find out why your thyroid is low, whether you have Hashimoto's, or your body is awash with too much prolactin.

This is a really important distinction, since excess levels of prolactin can actually be caused by tumors!

Thyroid Truth #10: Your TBG Could be too High

When your thyroid is humming along, happy as can be, it doesn't just release a single thyroid hormone. It releases three different hormones that each play their own important role in your body. These three thyroid hormones are:

- Triiodothyronine (T3)

- Tetraiodothyronine (T4)

- Calcionin

When your thyroid releases T3 and T4, they bind to a carrier protein called thyroxine-binding globulin. The name doesn't exactly roll off the tongue, which is why it is more commonly known as TBG. The TBG is like a limousine for your T3 and T4 hormones. When the TBG is working correctly, it drives T3 and T4 over to the liver for some important calibration and then drives them around the rest of the body wherever they are needed.

At some point, the T3 and T4 need to exit the limo so they can do their job of helping to regulate your metabolism. A problem can occur when there are too many limos on the road. If you have an elevated level of TBG in your system, it acts like thousands or millions of limos on the road, sucking up your T3 and T4 hormones, so that there aren't any free hormones to do what thyroid hormones are supposed to do. Everyone is stuck in a big limo traffic jam instead!

This situation can lead to hypothyroidism. Even worse, your blood tests may come back completely normal. After all, your thyroid is working just fine. It's just that your T3 and T4 are being kidnapped by the TBG. Some doctors may order blood tests to look at your T3 and T4. Even when the panels reveal that the level of these hormones in your system is low, they won't tell the doctor why the hormones are low. You need to find a doctor who will order a more detailed blood panel that looks at your level of TBG. Only then will any TBG issues come to light.

If you are wondering how the TBG can get so out of whack, one of the most common causes of elevated TBG is high levels of estrogen in the body. If you take birth control pills, or even use certain face creams or cosmetics that contain estrogen, you may be unknowingly raising your TBG levels, which could trap your thyroid hormones and leave you with symptoms of hypothyroidism.

Make sure you get the proper tests, so your medical professional can figure out what is truly going on in your body and where your symptoms are coming from.

Thyroid Truth #11: You Can't Treat Your Thyroid Until Your Blood Sugar is Under Control

Let's say that you have always dreamed of swimming

the English Channel. One day, you decide to go for it! You put on your bathing suit, strap on your goggles, and make sure your water wings are properly inflated. Ready to go!

Wait a minute…you can't possibly hope to swim the English Channel if you can't swim! Before you even dip your toe in the English Channel, it's time to head to the shallow end of your nearest neighborhood pool and start working on your doggy paddle and breast stroke.

This same thinking applies when we focus on improving the functionality of your thyroid to eliminate the symptoms of hypothyroidism. Before we can even begin to see big improvements in your thyroid, we must first get your blood sugar levels under control.

You need blood sugar (also known as glucose) to survive, just like you need fat in your body to survive. Blood sugar travels through your bloodstream and provides energy to your cells, which allows them to do all the wondrous things they do to keep you alive.

Our body is normally pretty good at balancing blood sugar levels, but that assumes we eat the right foods. We Americans are known to splurge, skip meals, and indulge in high-calorie, sugar-dense foods like fast food burgers, fries, and shakes. When our bodies are drowned in sugar, it becomes extremely difficult for our bodies to balance the blood sugar. As a result, blood sugar can rise to unhealthy levels in the body and cause all sorts of problems.

When fasting blood sugar rises above 127 mg/dL, the individual is considered to have diabetes. There is so much blood sugar in the body that the cells cannot absorb it all. According to the American Diabetes Association, 25.8 million people in the United States have diabetes, and a stunning 79 million people are considered pre-diabetic, which means that their blood sugar levels are on the precipice of being diabetic.

Type 2 diabetes, which accounts for approximately 90% of all cases of diabetes worldwide, is strongly related to lifestyle choices. Those who develop type 2 diabetes tend to have poor dietary habits and perform little regular exercise.

Receiving a diagnosis of diabetes or pre-diabetes can be a scary or overwhelming experience, but it can also act like a big push in the right direction. Changing your diet and your exercise patterns can create amazing changes in your body and help you reduce or even eliminate some of the symptoms that have been plaguing you for years!

Here's just one small but incredibly important tip for those with high blood sugar or who are hypoglycemic: Eat protein for breakfast, not carbohydrates. You need to eat eggs and lean meat such as turkey bacon for breakfast in order to support healthy blood sugar levels.

Even if your stomach feels upset in the morning, you still need to eat at least a little breakfast high in protein. This will likely help settle your stomach. If, after you get your blood levels under control, you still suffer symptoms like fatigue, low libido, and thinning hair, it may be time to look at your thyroid function.

Thyroid Truth #12: A Healthy Brain Makes a Healthy Thyroid

Just like in a natural ecosystem, if one part of your body starts slowing down or speeding up, it will create a ripple effect. For instance, if your estrogen levels spike, your TGB will also increase and will soak up T3 and T4 thyroid hormones like a sponge. Without T3 and T4 to help regulate your metabolism, you may feel tired and weak and notice weight gain.

No organ, hormone, or chemical inside your body works in a vacuum, especially not your thyroid. The brain plays a huge role in how your thyroid functions and whether or not it is healthy. Three parts of your brain that have the biggest impact on your thyroid are the pituitary gland, the neurotransmitter serotonin, and the hypothalamic periventricular nucleus. Let's take a brief look at how each works.

The Pituitary Gland

This pea-sized gland is tucked away in the center of the skull and releases many hormones, including thyroid stimulating hormone (TSH). TSH stimulates the thyroid to create thyroid hormone. If the pituitary gland doesn't release enough TSH, the thyroid puts up its feet and takes a nap. As a result, you suffer hypothyroidism. If the pituitary gland releases too much TSH, your thyroid goes into overdrive, and you find yourself with a case of hyperthyroidism.

Serotonin and hypothalamic periventricular nucleus

You probably know serotonin as the "feel-good" chemical, but it actually has a wide variety of functions in the digestive tract and central nervous system. This neurotransmitter acts on the hypothalamic periventricular nucleus, which in turn affects the level of TSH in your body.

If any of these three parts of your brain – the pituitary gland, serotonin, or hypothalamic periventricular nucleus – is out of whack, your thyroid will also become dysfunctional. This is a pretty big problem, especially since the normal synthetic thyroid hormones your doctor prescribes won't help fix your brain.

How Do You Fix Your Brain?

This leads to the obvious question, "So how exactly am I supposed to fix my brain if it has started slacking off?"

This is a big question that deserves much more than I can give in this quick guide. I can tell you that blood sugar is the biggest influencer on serotonin. If you suffer from hypoglycemia, insulin-resistance, or diabetes, you must address these issues and get your blood sugar levels into optimal range before you can hope to see big changes in your hypothyroid symptoms. The best way to manage your blood sugar is to change unhealthy habits. Kick your junk food habit to the curb and make regular exercise a part of your life.

Another big issue is oxygen. Both glucose and oxygen fuel your brain. If your brain doesn't receive optimal levels of oxygen, none of its parts, including the pituitary gland, can operate at its best level. (It's like running with a rubber mask over your face.) After the age of 25, your body's ability to utilize oxygen slowly begins to decrease. By the age of 50, you may be 25% less efficient at using oxygen than you were at age 25, which impacts how well the brain can function.

Certain oxygen therapies exist, and I provide clients with a special therapy called "Exercise with Oxygen Therapy." I encourage you to research and explore oxygen therapies available in your area.

Thyroid Truth #13: Gluten Could be the Culprit Behind Your Hypothyroidism

You may have heard about the gluten-free diet craze that is attracting celebrities, sport stars, and your neighbors to toss their gluten foods onto the proverbial bonfire. What is gluten? Why are so many people avoiding it, and what does it have to do with your thyroid?

Gluten is a protein found in wheat, barley, and rye. It's the stuff that gives dough its elasticity and makes bread, brownies, and cookies nice and chewy. Anything that contains flour or bread also contains gluten. It also shows up in all sorts of things you might not imagine, like soups and salad dressings.

Certain people, like me, suffer from celiac disease and cannot eat gluten because it causes inflammation in the small intestine. Only a small percentage of the population has celiac disease, but that's not the only reason gluten is dangerous.

We know that Hashimoto's disease is an autoimmune condition that causes the immune system to mistake thyroid hormones for intruders and unleash an immune response. The result is that your own immune system attacks your thyroid, wearing it down until it produces less and less of the thyroid hormones you need.

What causes the immune system to make this

mistake and attack the thyroid? These triggers are called **antigens**. A number of foods can function as antigens to certain people. Some of the more common are milk, soy, eggs, and yeast. By far the most common antigen is gluten. The structure of gluten is very similar to the structure of thyroid hormones. When gluten enters the body of someone with an autoimmune disorder, the immune system goes on the attack. In the midst of the battle frenzy, the white blood cells – the soldiers of the immune system – don't exactly stop to check to make sure they only attack gluten. They attack anything that looks like gluten, including thyroid hormones and the thyroid!

How do you know whether or not you are sensitive to gluten? There are tests available to check for a gluten allergy. At Labbe Health Center, we have a special relationship with an advanced lab that provides this testing to our clients. The lab doesn't just analyze blood samples, it actually takes a DNA swab (since we know that autoimmunity is genetic).

Once a client sends in their cheek swabs, they'll receive test results that let them know if you are sensitive to gluten, as well as other well-known antigens, like eggs, milk, yeast, and soy.

At last they know what's been causing all of their symptoms – why they always feels so tired, have trouble concentrating, and haven't felt cuddly and sexy for so long. The next step is removing identified antigens from the diet, so the immune system has no reason to attack the body.

At the end of this short book, I'll include my contact information if you are interested in learning more about this special lab and getting tested for food sensitivities.

Thyroid Truth #14: You Probably Need More Vitamin D

I know, I know, each time you pick up a women's health magazine the cover shouts about a new vitamin you absolutely must take. You'll also likely find a story about a previously popular vitamin that has been ejected from the cool kids table.

Vitamin D is here to stay. This vitamin is absolutely vital for healthy bones, healthy cells, and a strong immune system. In previous sections, I've told you what not to take to manage hypothyroidism. (No iodine or tyrosine!) Now it's time to tell you what can help your condition.

Vitamin D is one of the best vitamins you can take if you have hypothyroidism. It also happens that very few people get enough Vitamin D in their diets. Actually, as rates of Vitamin D in the average person have gone down, rates of hypothyroidism have skyrocketed. Coincidence?

You can get Vitamin D in three primary ways: through your food, through absorption of sunlight, and through supplements. You can find Vitamin D in liver, organ meats, lard, some seafood, and egg yolks. If you don't have a big, steaming plate of liver or lard around (Yuck!), you can also stand outside and let Vitamin D from the sun absorb through your skin. If you're more of the indoor type, then a Vitamin D supplement is probably your best bet.

Why is Vitamin D so important? We've found that Vitamin D deficiency is associated with many autoimmune conditions, including Hashimoto's disease. Some research has shown that a large majority of the people with an autoimmune thyroid or Hashimoto's also have a genetic defect that messes with their ability to process Vitamin D.

Adequate Vitamin D levels help to keep the immune system in balance so it doesn't swing out of control into an autoimmune disease

Tests can be performed to determine the level of Vitamin D in your body. Many doctors will only perform a single test to look for 25-hydroxyvitamin D (25-OHD). I strongly recommend looking at two different factors, 25-OHD and 125-OHD for a clearer picture of your Vitamin D levels.

I believe that the current medical standards of "normal" Vitamin D levels are overly broad. Your tests may show that your Vitamin D level is on the low side of "normal", but I don't think "normal" is good enough. I want your Vitamin D level to be optimal, which is why I often suggest Vitamin D supplements to my clients if they have an autoimmune condition. Another thing I strongly recommend for clients is essential fatty acids.

Thyroid Truth #15: Essential Fatty Acids (EFAs) are Your Friends

America has had an on-again, off-again relationship with dietary fats. For years, you couldn't walk through a grocery store aisle without passing bags, boxes, and cartons proudly announcing low-fat treats within.

Most consumers today realize that there is more than one fat and that certain fats are essential to a person's health and well-being. When you hear the latest obesity statistics, you may be convinced that we Americans are eating too much fat. The problem is a little more complex.

Fats are Good for You

Omega 6 and Omega 3 fatty acids are the building blocks of healthy cells, a healthy brain, and a healthy nervous system. Our bodies cannot create these fats, so we must consume them in our food or through supplementation. Omega 6 fatty acids come from plant oils, like corn oil and sunflower oil, as well as nuts and seeds. Omega 3 fatty acids are found in fatty fish like salmon, mackerel, and tuna, as well as walnuts and flaxseed. Many who cannot steam fish for dinner every day choose to take fish oil pills to get their daily dose of Omega 3.

If life were simple, then you could simply eat as much

Omega 6 and Omega 3 fatty acids as you wanted and enjoy abundant health. Unfortunately, our bodies are not so straightforward. In fact, your good health doesn't just depend on how much Omega 6 and Omega 3 fatty acids you consume, but the ratio of the two different fats. Research suggests that you should consume a ratio of 3 to 1 up to 5 to 1 of Omega 6 vs. Omega 3.

So far, we Americans haven't gotten the memo. The Standard American Diet (appropriately known as S.A.D.) contains a ratio of 25 to 1 Omega 6 fatty acids vs. Omega 3 fatty acids. This lopsided teeter totter is a big reason behind all the, well, BIG Americans we see waddling around.

Our SAD Diet

The Standard American Diet truly is SAD. Count the number of fast food restaurants you pass on your way to work, count the calories on the average menu, and look around to see how many people are guzzling soft drinks at any local gathering. Our diets are filled with junk!

Consider your diet over the last two weeks. Have you been putting lots of junk into your body? Those are the same materials your body will use to build new cells, feed your brain, and energize your body. If half of what you eat comes out of a box, or is covered in sugar and hot fudge, your body just won't have good building materials to keep you healthy.

If you are serious about correcting your thyroid problem and becoming a healthier person, then you need to change your diet and focus on balancing your ratio of fats. No excuses. Get rid of the junk food and start taking essential fatty acids.

Thyroid Truth #16: Polycystic Ovarian Syndrome Can Lead to Hashimoto's

A healthy body is truly a balanced body. Beneath the confines of your skin, a precious ecosystem exists filled with hormones, sugars, fats, organs, bacteria, and flora that all affect each other. If even one part of the ecosystem gets out of balance, it can slowly poison the entire system.

A good example of this concept is Polycystic Ovarian Syndrome, PCOS. According to WomensHealth.gov, as many as 1 in 10 women of childbearing age could have PCOS. This condition gets its name from the small cysts present on an affected woman's ovaries.

The symptoms of PCOS are not pretty:

- Acne

- Weight gain

- Excessive hair growth

- Missed or irregular periods

- Infertility

- Anxiety and depression

What causes PCOS, and more importantly, how can we avoid it? The medical community isn't exactly sure what causes PCOS, but there does seem to be a genetic component. If your mother or sister suffers from PCOS, then you are more likely to develop the condition as well.

Hormonal imbalance plays a big role in PCOS. One hallmark of the condition is higher-than-usual levels of androgen, a male sex hormone. The androgen causes lovely side effects like acne and excess hair. It also lowers the production of progesterone, a hormone that regulates the menstrual cycle and supports fertility.

As we learned in a previous article, a deficiency in progesterone can lead to an increase in prolactin, which stresses out the pituitary gland and causes it to release less thyroid stimulating hormone. You can see how one fluctuating hormone triggers a change in another and another, and another, until the entire body starts to fall to pieces. PCOS sufferers often develop insulin resistance, which can cause blood sugar levels to skyrocket and increase the risk of diabetes.

PCOS can also trigger your immune system to go on a rampage. The thyroid is a likely target of an autoimmune response. Over time, you could develop Hashimoto's disease, where your immune system attacks your thyroid.

All too often, doctors will simply prescribe synthetic hormones to patients suffering from hypothyroidism. This strategy might alleviate symptoms, but it completely ignores the cause – the big picture of your body's ecosystem.

Instead of just swallowing a thyroid pill every day, women need to test for PCOS among many other possibilities. Only once your progesterone and androgen hormones are back in balance can you begin to help balance out the rest of your body, including your thyroid.

Thyroid Truth #17: Stress Could be Strangling Your Thyroid

How are you feeling right now? Does the word "stressed" come to mind? If you're like many Americans, you have a long to-do list constantly scrolling through the back of your mind. You spend your days racing to get your children to soccer and gymnastic practice, dueling it out with other cars on the highway, puzzling through the latest criticism from your passive-aggressive coworker, paying the mortgage, fixing the latest thing to break, and scrolling through work email even at night when you're supposed to be relaxing.

Whew! I feel a bit stressed just writing all of that. The truth is, our modern society is highly conducive to stress. Not just any kind of stress – low grade chronic stress. I think of it as a weighted vest constantly slowing our steps, keeping us at a standstill.

We all know that stress causes gray hair, wrinkles, and even dangerous symptoms, like high blood pressure and ulcers. That's because stress is like an explosive domino, triggering all sorts of chaos in our body, including suppression of the thyroid.

It all starts with two innocuous seeming glands, one atop each kidney. These adrenal glands may be small, but they are each a veritable treasure chest of hormones. When they get humming, they unleash cortisol, aldosterone, testosterone, epinephrine, and norepinephrine, just to name a few. These powerful hormones, especially cortisol, can cause big changes in the body.

Stress has always been part of life, whether it comes from a charging saber tooth tiger a hundred thousand years ago or a truck running a red light in the intersection this morning. When we find ourselves in a stressful situation, the adrenal glands kick into high gear, pouring hormones into our system. You've no doubt been in a frightening situation where you felt your heart rate double and every sense in your body heighten. Your body was jacked with energy, strength, and focus, allowing you to flee, fight, or respond immediately to the threat (even if that meant just slamming on your brakes to avoid an accident).

This is what the stress response is supposed to do. It can save your life or help you avoid injury during emergency situations. However, the adrenal glands haven't had the chance to evolve in the age of all-night college cram sessions, job interviews, endless traffic, or the requirements of modern parenting. Our adrenals can't tell the difference between the non-threatening-yet-stressful situation of waiting in line at the DMV and the truly dangerous situation of facing a rattle snake on a hiking trail.

When a woman experiences chronic stress, her adrenal glands are working overtime, filling her body with a toxic mix of hormones, including cortisol, which can lead to weight gain and insulin resistance. Your adrenals also release a small protein called cytokines, which suppresses the pituitary gland (more on cytokines next). Remember, your pituitary gland is a small gland in the brain that creates thyroid stimulating hormone (TSH), which tells your thyroid to get to work. Low levels of TSH mean that your thyroid will go on vacation, leading to hypothyroidism.

If the chronic stress continues for years or even decades (not uncommon!), the adrenal glands may actually exhaust themselves, like a car engine worn down by 200,000 miles of hard driving. This results in a whole host of additional problems that also affect the thyroid.

High levels of cortisol can also be caused by post-traumatic stress disorder, gut infections, and even parasites, but the most common cause is stress, stress, and more stress!

We all know that we need to manage the stress in our lives, but hopefully when you realize how much it messes with your body, you'll have an even bigger incentive to kick the stressors out of your life and treat yourself with more self-love and care.

Thyroid Truth #18: Small Protein Messengers May be Shutting Off Your Thyroid

The human body is amazingly complex. On the microscopic level, you are filled with thousands of proteins, hormones, cells, and other compounds whizzing by, all working to keep you "out and about" and feeling great.

A group of small proteins that play an important role inside your body are called cytokines. Haven't heard of them before? That's normal. Cytokines don't often get the spotlight, even though they could be part of the reason you feel so blah every day.

Think of cytokines as the molecular Pony Express, galloping through your body and telling certain cells what to do, especially when it comes to your inflammatory response.

If you have an inflammatory condition like arthritis, IBS, asthma, or an autoimmune condition like lupus or rheumatoid arthritis, you probably have lots of cytokines rushing around delivering important messages.

Unfortunately, cytokines aren't always benign little messengers. When cytokine levels get high, they can actually suppress the function of the pituitary gland in the brain. As we learned earlier, the pituitary gland is a pea-shaped gland in the brain that produces thyroid stimulating hormone, TSH. TSH gives the "giddy-up" to your thyroid so it produces thyroid hormone and keeps you riding high.

When cytokines suppress the pituitary, it doesn't release enough TSH, and your thyroid goes out to pasture. A low functioning thyroid results in hypothyroidism and all the wonderful symptoms you have come to know and love, like weight gain, thinning hair, exhaustion, brain fog, dry skin, and low libido.

So, how do we get you on some happier trails? My motto is, "Testing, not guessing." When I start working with clients, I suggest a variety blood and fluids tests, including a test for different types of cytokines. If I see high levels of a particular cytokine, it's likely that the client's pituitary gland is taking a snooze along with their thyroid.

Again, if you are interested in learning more about the tests I suggest for my clients or the third party labs that I use, please contact me for more information.

Thyroid Truth #19: Improving Your Intestinal Fortitude Can Improve Your Thyroid Function

Did you know that your gut can actually leak? It sounds yucky, but it's true! For those who suffer from "Leaky Gut Syndrome" (LGS), the lining of their intestine has become so permeable that food particles and large molecules can actually slip out into the body and blood stream.

Can you imagine tiny bits of your dinner floating around in your body? LGS causes all sorts of chaos inside your body. It also revs up the immune system, which must hunt down and eliminate all those stray particles.

A healthy GI tract is a tight mesh of tissue that keeps bacteria, digested food, and other particles inside the gut and out of the blood stream. Chronic inflammation is a main cause of LGS, as are parasites. I know exactly what you're saying to yourself, "I haven't been wandering around the rainforest drinking from dirty streams, so of course I don't have parasites!"

You'd be surprised at how easy it is to get a parasite, even in the middle of USA suburbia. Many of my clients are surprised when we discover parasites in their system.

Inflammation is a gut destroyer! It's also a self-replicating cycle. When you suffer from LGS, every time you eat, particles wiggled through the weak lining of your intestines into the bloodstream, triggering an immune system red alert. This happens every single time you eat. Additionally, it also causes a huge amount of inflammation, which further weakens the gut.

This constant cycle of inflammation and immune system response sets the stage for an autoimmune condition, like Hashimoto's disease. Even as the immune system is trying to mop up all the stray particles leaking out of your gut, it may also start attacking your thyroid, causing hypothyroidism.

This is a lot to think about, I know, but if you imagine your body as a delicate ecosystem, you'll understand how one small problem can snowball into chronic health conditions.

So, how do we tighten up a leaky gut? The solution isn't as easy as plugging a hole with Gorilla Glue. First, you must stop the cycle of inflammation so that your gut can actually begin repairing itself. That means you must stop eating the foods that commonly cause an inflammatory response. The five biggest culprits are: gluten, soy, milk, eggs, and yeast.

When I discover that a client has a leaky gut, I immediately put her on a 4R colon program, which entails eliminating gluten, soy, milk, eggs, and yeast from the diet, getting parasites out of the body, inoculating against future parasites, and using probiotics to build back up healthy flora in the gut. This regimen has done wonders for my clients. Many times, simply repairing the gut can reduce or even completely eliminate their symptoms of hypothyroidism. If the immune system doesn't have to be on red alert all the time, it will have less reason to attack the thyroid.

Thyroid Truth #20: You Aren't Crazy, Lazy, or Finished, No Matter What Your Doctor Tells You!

There is nothing quite as frustrating as a "normal" test result when you're feeling lousy. You know something is wrong, even though your doctor tells you that your blood tests are normal.

Yeah right! You feel exhausted every day, like you've got sandbags strapped to your ankles. You used to be great at remembering dates, but your mind's so foggy that you wouldn't be surprised if you forgot your own birthday. You never feel like you're in the mood to be intimate, and you toss and turn at night no matter how tired you feel.

This isn't normal! Yet, after the third doctor shakes her head and tells you that you are fine, it's tempting to believe that it's all in your head, that you're being overdramatic, or that this is what it feels like to grow older. Your family members and friends may even start to wonder if you're going crazy.

I cannot count how many women have come into my office after having seen multiple doctors who all say they are fine. These women are desperate for answers and desperate to find out that they aren't just making it up.

They aren't and neither are you! Most primary care physicians run only a basic blood panel, which gives them a limited amount of information. Additionally, doctors look for results that indicate serious illness. If your numbers aren't in catastrophic ranges, they consider you to be "normal".

There's that word again. Normal does not mean healthy. In fact, you can experience symptoms even though you are not yet ill enough to raise red flags as far as your doctor is concerned. This is the difference between a traditional medicine approach and a functional medicine approach.

Functional medicine focuses on identifying health issues even in their early stages and helping clients regain optimal health. There is a world of difference between the word "optimal" and the word "normal."

A doctor may consider a normal level of Thyroid Stimulating Hormone to be between .35 – 5.0. If you're in this range, your doctor will probably say that you are perfectly fine. I'm not looking for a normal TSH level. I look to see if your TSH level is within optimal range, which is 1.8 – 3.0. If you are outside of this range, you may be normal, but you certainly aren't in optimal health.

Additionally, one simple blood test isn't enough. If your TSH is low, then we need to figure out why. Are you having an autoimmune response? Is your gut leaking? Are you experiencing an inflammatory response to gluten, milk, soy, eggs, or yeast? Do you have a parasite?

To answer these questions, we need to run multiple tests on your blood and fluids. Information truly is power, and your thyroid specialist needs as much information as possible to help you develop a treatment plan to manage or eliminate the cause of your hypothyroid symptoms.

Don't ever let a doctor make you feel like you are "Lazy, Crazy, or Finished." If you feel terrible every day, then your body is trying to tell you that something isn't right.

Thyroid Truth #21: A Diagnosis is Just the Beginning

It can be scary when your body is out of whack and you don't know why. You feel the symptoms. You suffer. You know something isn't right. But without an answer – without a name – you are helpless to find relief.

When your doctor finally puts a name to your symptoms, like "hypothyroidism" or "anemia," you might hear a mini choir of angels in your mind singing *Hallelujah*! You aren't crazy. There really is something wrong that your doctor can fix!

I understand the relief in receiving a diagnosis, especially if you have been suffering with symptoms for months or even years. I went through the same thing before I discovered I had celiac disease. I felt "off," but I didn't know why until I tested myself and saw the telltale results.

As nice as it is to have a name for your condition, don't let a label lull you into a false sense of security. Hypothyroidism, for example, simply refers to the fact that your thyroid is not releasing enough thyroid hormone. Many different things can cause hypothyroidism. In this book I've explained many of the different causes of hypothyroidism, like Hashimoto's, leaky gut, and sensitivity to gluten. We've also learned that certain conditions can play on each other. For instance, a sensitivity to gluten could lead to inflammation, which could lead to a leaky gut, which could lead to an autoimmune response, which could lead to hypothyroidism.

When it comes to hypothyroidism, a label is only the beginning. It is like a flare in the night sky, showing us where we need to start looking for the causes of the low thyroid. Many traditional primary care practitioners will see low thyroid function on your blood test and prescribe you synthetic thyroid hormones. This may temporarily relieve some of your symptoms, but it's like taking out the batteries of a fire alarm. It doesn't actually put out the fire, it just stops your body from making noise.

Functional medicine seeks to help clients reach optimal health through extensive testing and retesting. It's not enough to determine that you have low thyroid function. You need to find out if you are also having an autoimmune reaction, if you test positive for food allergies, if any parasites are in your gut, and a number of other things.

Once you start a treatment plan, then you must retest to see if you are actually getting better. Is your thyroid hormone production increasing? Does your thyroid specialist see a lower level of antibodies in your bloods, which indicates that your immune system is settling down? Are your markers showing less inflammation, suggesting that your gut is beginning to heal? Do you actually feel better?

A diagnosis is only the beginning.

Thyroid Truth #22: Don't Just Take the Batteries Out of the Fire Alarm

We can all agree that the sound of a fire alarm is not pleasant, but fire alarms serve a very important purpose. They let us know that something is wrong. If you woke up in the middle of the night and heard the fire alarm going off, would you take the batteries out of the alarm and go back to bed?

No! You would look for the fire and put it out!

When you feel lousy for weeks, months, or even years, your body is trying to tell you that something is wrong. If you are constipated, tired, or can't remember your children's birthdays, that's your body's fire alarm.

Medication can be a huge relief, but it can also be a crutch. You could just be taking the batteries out of the fire alarm without putting out the fire.

If your doctor discovers that your thyroid is underactive, she will likely prescribe synthetic thyroid hormones. This medicine may temporarily help relieve some of your symptoms (although, in some cases it won't even do that!), but it is just a crutch. Something is causing your thyroid to stop producing the hormones your body needs. Instead of fixing the cause (putting out the fire), the medicine will simply address the symptoms. In most cases, whatever is causing the issue will get worse, and your doctor will simply increase your dosage year by year.

There are certain situations where medication is critical for health and relief, and I am not suggesting that you throw all your medicine away today. I am simply saying that it is easy to become reliant on medicine instead of tackling the underlying issues.

I can't tell you how many people I've seen who started off with one or two medications in their thirties, ended up with four or five medications in their fifties, and now take thirteen to fifteen medications in their eighties. I'm sure you have friends or family members who fit this very stereotype.

When it comes to low thyroid function, it is highly possible that, through testing, that a trained thyroid specialist can help you figure out what's causing the problem. Together, you can then determine a natural treatment plan to help fix the issue(s). It may be as simple as taking gluten out of your diet or getting rid of parasites in your gut. As you improve, you may come to a point where you can go back to your doctor and ask her to decrease your thyroid medication or take you off of it altogether.

Thyroid Truth #23: Embrace Your Body as an Ecosystem

If you've read this far, then I bet you can fill in the missing blank.

Your body is like its own....

Ecosystem!

Your body is an incredibly complex place, filled with many different chemicals that all exist within a precarious balance. If even one hormone or protein level gets too high or too low, it can trigger a domino effect that sends your body into a tailspin. That's why so many diseases like hypothyroidism, Hashimoto's, and Grave's disease present with a wide range of symptoms. It's not just one thing going wrong in your body; many different things are out of whack. Your ecosystem is out of balance.

Traditional medicine is really good at treating emergency situations, like a broken bone, stroke, or traumatic injuries from a car crash. Doctors can see the broken bone in an X-ray, set it, and wrap a cast on it. There, problem solved!

They have more trouble with chronic conditions where symptoms come from all over the body and have many different causes. You can't just set a broken bone when it comes to Hashimoto's. You must determine what factors are affecting the thyroid and why those things are acting up. In many cases, you begin to find a chain reaction. A leaky gut leads to inflammation, which leads to an autoimmune response, which leads to a suppressed thyroid.

Chronic conditions require a practitioner to look at the whole person. This is big picture treatment that often involves lots of different testing, a multi-step treatment plan, and constant tweaking and retesting to assess changes to the individual.

I've just described the basis of functional medicine. You've heard this term a lot in this book. Functional medicine is predicated upon the use of thorough testing and natural remedies to help individuals achieve optimal health.

Many post-menopausal women are suffering and they don't know why. They feel like their bodies are breaking down. In many cases, the reason has to do with low thyroid functioning. Too many of these women go to the doctor's office only to be told that their tests are normal. They leave thinking that they are lazy, crazy, and finished!

You are not lazy, crazy, and finished. You simply haven't gone to the right authority yet.

Thyroid Truth #24: You're Either Getting Better or Worse

Many people believe that as long as they are not sick, they are well, as if wellness were some type of static condition or a line in the sand that can be crossed. Reality is much more complicated, and I hope you have started to develop a more nuanced understanding of health as a result of this book.

Your body is an ecosystem. Every choice that you make is a choice toward health or a choice toward sickness. Tomorrow morning, you can choose to eat a protein-rich breakfast or you can choose to skip breakfast altogether. You can choose to accept the passive aggressive behavior of your coworker or confront her and air your issues. You can choose to eat Doritos for lunch or order a salad. You can choose to run three miles in the evening or watch a marathon of *Storage Wars* on the couch.

You get the picture. Every choice you make pushes you in one direction or the other. You might not feel the effects of a skipped breakfast, a stressful work environment, or an evening of vegging on the couch tomorrow, but they have a cumulative effect. Ever so slowly, poor choices can push you over the edge into sickness, where you begin to feel real symptoms.

Here's another choice you can make – you can choose to rely on medicine for the rest of your life to control your hypothyroid symptoms, or you can choose to find out what's causing the symptoms in the first place.

When you understand what is causing your illness, you're presented with another choice, keep doing the same old things, or make the life changes that will help you feel better.

If you've stayed with me this far, then I think I know which choices you will make. Don't wait any longer. Change can be scary, I know, but it can also lead to wondrous discoveries. I can't think of a better discovery than the feeling of true health, especially after years of feeling crazy, lazy, and finished. Make the right choice and start taking actions that honor your body and protect your health.

Thyroid Truth #25: You Are in Charge of Your Health Destiny

The purpose of this book is to reveal truths about your thyroid condition. Here's a hard truth that often gets lost in all the talk about hormones and proteins and different glands of the body: Nobody is going to care about you more than you.

You and only you are responsible for your health. Many of the chronic illnesses that plague our society, like diabetes, heart disease, and even certain forms of cancer are related to the lifestyle decisions that we make. Even when we can't avoid an illness, like gluten sensitivity or celiac disease, we can control how we manage it.

We can choose to ignore symptoms, we can give up when a doctor tells us that we're fine, or we can keep pushing for answers! We can also choose to just treat our symptoms with medication or to try and improve our condition by fixing the underlying causes.

With something as complex as hypothyroidism, Hashimoto's thyroiditis, or Grave's disease, you have to literally grab the bull by the horns and take charge. That means extensive testing to figure out exactly what is going wrong in the body so that we can come up with a treatment plan. My functional medicine approach has taught me to try to use natural means to heal imbalances in the body, often through changes in diet and lifestyle.

In some cases, especially in the case of serious illness or trauma, medicine is truly the best approach, but in other instances I believe that we can help the body heal itself just by taking care of it the right way.

As for you, if something (or everything) doesn't feel right, then it's up to you to take action. Don't let a doctor tell you that you are normal. Don't think a prescription is the only option for your health woes. I challenge you to do better for yourself.

It's Time to Take Action

My fabulous friend, we've reached the end of this short book, but I hope we're at the very beginning of your journey back to health. This book was only a start – a quick guide to help you understand *what* is happening inside your body and *why* your doctor may not have all the answers and solutions that you need.

I have so much more that I want to share with you! I know you must have many questions, like:

- How do I find out if I have an autoimmune condition?

- What type of tests do I really need and how do I get them?

- How can I interpret these tests, or where can I find someone who can?

- What can I change in my diet right now to start feeling better?

I can offer you several different ways to get the answers you need. If you enjoyed reading this book, then I strongly suggest my much bigger and more detailed follow-up, *Why Is Mid-Life Mooching Your Mojo?* available as an ebook, paperback, and hardback on Amazon.com. In *Why Is Mid-Life Mooching Your Mojo?*, I expand on everything we just learned about in this book and take it to the next level by showing you exactly how you can regain your health using completely natural methods. This volume is packed with great information, most of it things your doctor will never tell you!

If you want more direct guidance and coaching, or if you have any questions as a result of this book, please reach out to me. I continue to selectively take on private clients and offer several different levels of coaching. I can review your case with you directly, develop a testing protocol just for you, and guide you to a private lab in your area to have your testing done. The results will be mind-blowing, I promise! We'll review them together to actually see what is going on inside your body, which will help me design a wellness plan that will change your life. To schedule a consultation, please contact me at support@mojogirlfriends.com .

And finally, I want you to know that you don't have to go through this struggle alone. Too often, middle-aged women feel overlooked and forgotten. You are gorgeous and wonderful and deserving of love and attention! I invite you to visit my special online community, www.mojogirlfriends.com where you can share your story, connect with other women, and where we can all support each other in our journey towards health and happiness. This is the place to ask those private questions that you're too embarrassed to ask your friends, learn more about the lessons in this book, and gain access to great new tools and resources that I will be adding to the site as the community grows. I have big plans for www.MojoGirlfriends.com, but I need your participation and enthusiasm to help this site grow!

Last but not least, if you found this book helpful, please take a moment to write and post a review on

Amazon and to share that review through social media if you feel comfortable. Thank you so much for your support, and I wish you an abundance of health, happiness, and love in your life!

Dr. Joni Labbe, DC, CCN, DCCN

Made in the USA
San Bernardino, CA
27 March 2015